JUICING FOR BEGINNERS

A STEP-BY-STEP GUIDE TO UNLOCKING THE BENEFITS OF JUICING AT HOME

Donna Williams

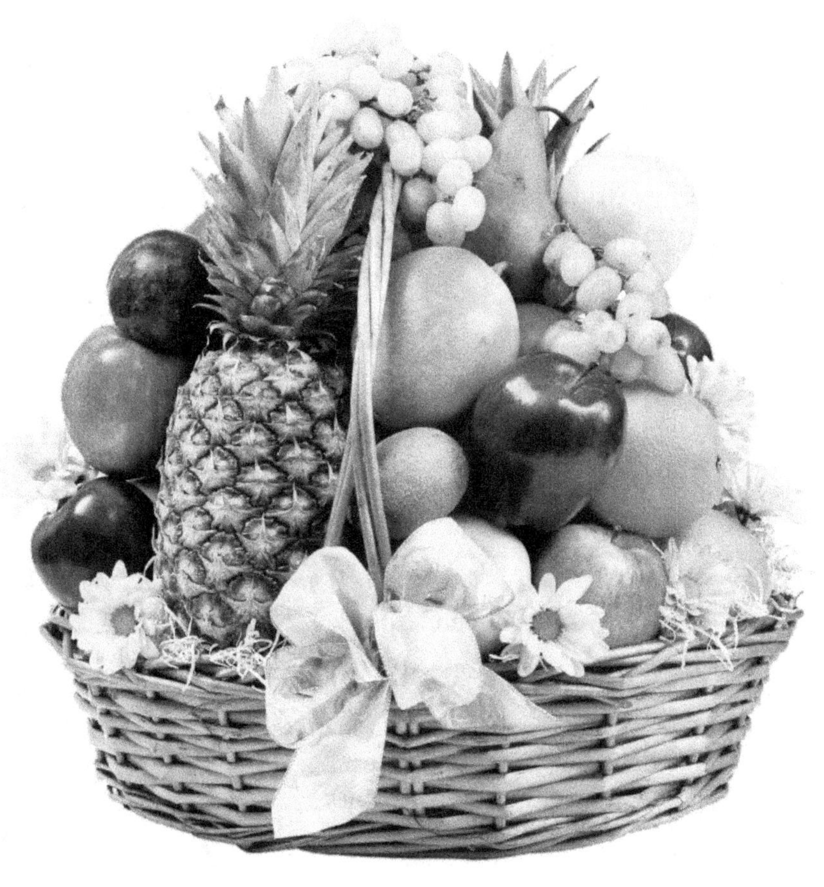

TABLE OF CONTENT

INTRODUCTION

Kevin had heard all the hype about juicing, but he was always skeptical. How could something as simple as blending fruits and vegetables together be so beneficial? He had to try it and find out for himself.

Kevin started slowly. He began with a basic mixture of carrots, apples, and oranges. He found that the flavor was delicious, and it seemed to give him more energy. He started to experiment with different combinations of fruits and vegetables, and soon he was hooked.

He was soon adding spinach, kale, and other leafy greens to his recipes. He also began to use turmeric, ginger, and other spices to give his juice an extra boost of flavor.

As he began to drink more of his homemade juices, Kevin noticed a difference. He felt healthier and more energetic. His skin was glowing and he was feeling less sluggish.

After a few months, Kevin's friends and family started to take notice. They asked him what he was doing differently and he proudly shared his juicing secrets. Soon they were all trying out his recipes and reaping the benefits.

Kevin continued to drink his juices every day and was soon living a much healthier lifestyle. He was able to maintain his weight, his energy levels were high, and he was even able to fight off colds and other illnesses.

After years of juicing, Kevin was still feeling great. He had more energy and vitality than ever before, and he was living a long and healthy life. He was thankful that he had taken the time to experiment with juicing and discover its amazing health benefits.

Juicing for Beginners is an essential guide for anyone looking to get started on a life-changing journey to better health through juicing. This book provides an in-depth look at the science behind why juicing works, as well as step-by-step instructions on how to create delicious, nutritious juice recipes. With easy-to-follow tips and suggestions, juicing for Beginners will teach you how to get the most out of your juicing experience, and help you become an expert in no time. Whether you're a beginner or an experienced juicer, this book will provide you with all the information you need to start creating delicious and nutritious juices that will fuel your body and energize your mind.

CHAPTER 1

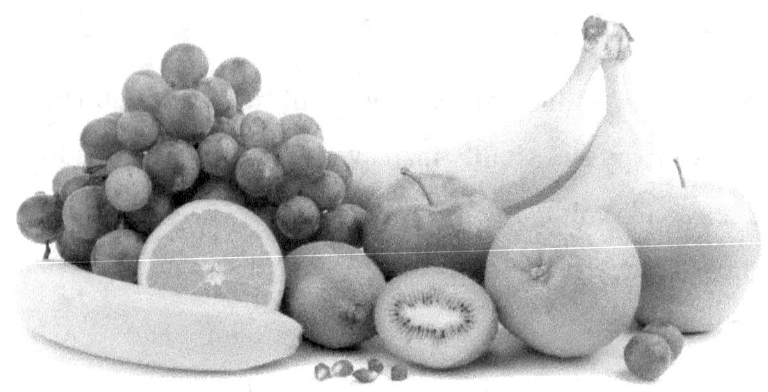

What is Juicing

Juicing is a process of extracting juice from fruits and vegetables in order to obtain their nutrients and other health benefits. Juicing is a popular health trend that has been gaining a lot of attention in recent years. The process involves using a juicer to mechanically extract juice from fruits and vegetables, leaving behind the pulp or fiber. Juicing provides a concentrated dose of vitamins, minerals, and other nutrients that are difficult to obtain from a typical diet. Additionally, it can help to detoxify the body, boost the immune system, increase energy levels, and aid in weight loss. Juicing is a great way to add more fruits and vegetables to your diet without having to eat them all in one sitting. It is also a convenient way to get your daily recommended servings of fruits and vegetables. However, it is important to note that juicing does not replace whole fruits and vegetables and should be used in addition to a balanced diet.

In addition, juicing entails a wide range of health benefits. It helps to increase nutrient absorption by breaking down the fruits and vegetables into a more easily digestible form. Juicing also helps to increase the bioavailability of certain vitamins and minerals, allowing them to be more readily absorbed by the body. Additionally, it can help to detoxify the body by removing toxins and impurities. Juicing can also help to boost the immune system and provide a concentrated dose of vitamins and minerals to support overall health. Finally, it can help to increase energy levels and aid in weight loss.

Benefits of Juicing

1. Improved Nutrition: Juicing provides a concentrated dose of vitamins, minerals, and other beneficial nutrients, such as

antioxidants and phytonutrients. This can help to ensure that you are getting the recommended daily intake of these essential nutrients.

2. Weight Loss: Juicing can be a great way to lose weight as it helps to reduce calorie intake while providing essential nutrients. The fiber in the juice helps to keep you feeling full for a longer period of time, helping to reduce cravings and overeating.

3. Cleansing: Juicing can help to flush toxins from the body, as the fresh juice is rich in vitamins, minerals and antioxidants.

4. Improved Digestion: Juicing helps to break down the fiber in the fruits and vegetables, making them easier to digest. This can help to reduce digestive issues, such as bloating and constipation.

5. Energy Boost: Juicing helps to provide an instant energy boost due to the concentrated nutrients. This can be great for those who need an extra boost of energy during the day.

6. Enhanced Skin Health: Juicing can help to improve skin health as it provides essential vitamins and minerals that can help to improve collagen production and skin elasticity.

7. Improved Immune System: Juicing can help to boost the immune system due to the high concentration of vitamins and minerals. This can help to reduce the risk of illness and disease.

Equipment Needed for Juicing

1. Juicer: A juicer is the most essential piece of equipment needed for juicing. Juicers come in many shapes and sizes, ranging from simple hand-held citrus juicers to high-end masticating juicers. Depending on the type of juicer you choose, some models can also be used for making nut milk and purees.

2. Blender: A blender is also a useful tool for juicing. Blenders can be used to juice soft fruits and vegetables, as well as to make creamy smoothies and soups.

3. Cutting Board: A cutting board is essential for prepping fruits and vegetables before juicing. It's important to use a cutting board to avoid cross-contamination of food.

4. Knife: A sharp knife is needed to cut fruits and vegetables into smaller pieces so that they can fit through the juicer's chute.

5. Strainer: A strainer can be used to separate the pulp from the juice. This is an optional step, but it can help to make a smoother, more enjoyable juice.

6. Bowls and Containers: Bowls and containers are needed to collect and store the juice. Glass jars or containers with lids are great for storing juice in the fridge.

7. Cleaning Supplies: Cleaning supplies such as a brush and detergent are necessary for cleaning the juicer and containers after each use.

Types of Juicers

There are many different types of juicers on the market today, each with its own unique design and features. Knowing the different types of juicers will help you decide which one is right for you.

Centrifugal Juicers: These are the most common type of juicers, and are typically the most affordable. They use a rapidly spinning metal blade to cut the fruit or vegetable into small pieces, releasing the juice. Centrifugal juicers are fast, efficient, and easy to use, but are not always the best at extracting the maximum amount of juice.

Masticating Juicers: Also known as "slow juicers", masticating juicers use an auger (or screw) to slowly crush and press the fruit or vegetable, releasing the juice in a very efficient manner. They are excellent for maximizing juice yield, but are usually more expensive and are usually louder than centrifugal juicers.

Triturating Juicers: These are the most advanced type of juicers, and are typically the most expensive. Triturating juicers use two augers that press the fruit or vegetable against a screen, releasing the juice. They are very efficient at extracting juice, and are the best option for leafy greens and wheatgrass.

Citrus Juicers: As the name implies, citrus juicers are specifically designed for juicing citrus fruits, such as lemons, limes, and oranges. They typically come in a manual or electric design, and use a reamer to press and extract the juice, making them fast and efficient.

Cold Press Juicers: Also known as "slow juicers", cold press juicers use a hydraulic press to slowly press and extract the juice from fruits and vegetables. They are excellent for maximizing nutrient retention and extracting the most juice, but they are quite expensive and usually require more effort to operate.

Other types of juicers include manual juicers, juice extractors, and blenders. Each type of juicer has its own unique design and features, and will suit different needs. Knowing the different types of juicers and what they can do will help you decide which type is best for you.

CHAPTER 2

Tips & Tricks

1. Choose fruits and vegetables that have the most nutritional benefits. Fruits and vegetables that are high in antioxidants and nutrients are best for juicing. Look for organic produce whenever possible.

2. Incorporate leafy greens such as spinach, kale, and Swiss chard as they are packed with vitamins, minerals, and other nutrients.

3. Use only organic lemons and limes for juicing as these have the highest vitamin C content.

4. Start juicing with mild and sweet fruits and vegetables such as apples, pears, and carrots before progressing to more bitter and pungent flavors.

5. Use a combination of fruits and vegetables for the best flavor and maximum nutritional benefit.

6. Add a small amount of ginger, garlic, or cayenne pepper for a spicy kick.

7. Use a slow speed juicer for the best nutrient extraction and minimal oxidation.

8. Drink your juice as soon as possible, as oxidation will degrade the nutritional value over time.

9. Store your juice in a sealed container in the refrigerator, and consume within 24 hours.

10. If you are using a centrifugal juicer, try to alternate between hard and soft ingredients to ensure the best extraction.

Choosing the Right Fruits and Vegetables

When it comes to juicing, it is important to choose the right fruits and vegetables for the best tasting juice and the most nutritional benefits. The following tips can help you make the most of your juicing experience.

First, be sure to select fruits and vegetables that are in season. This will help to ensure that you are getting the freshest produce with the highest nutritional value. You can find out what is in season in your area by checking the local grocery stores or farmers markets.

Second, select fruits and vegetables that are ripe. Unripe fruits and vegetables may not provide the same nutritional benefits as those that are ripe. Ripe produce also tastes better and can make your juice more enjoyable.

Third, consider your preferences and health goals when selecting fruits and vegetables. If you want a sweeter juice, select fruits like apples, oranges, and bananas. If you want a more savory juice, select vegetables like kale, spinach, and celery.

Finally, remember that with juicing you can always experiment. If you're feeling adventurous, try combining different fruits and vegetables to create a unique flavor. You may find that you like the taste of a combination that you would have never thought of on your own.

Storing Your Juices

When it comes to juicing, one of the most important things to consider is how to store your juices. Although homemade juices are very healthy and delicious, they can easily turn bad if not stored properly. Here are some tips to keep your juices fresh and tasty:

1. Refrigerate your juices as soon as possible. Fresh-squeezed juices are best consumed within 15 minutes of being made, however, if you can't drink it right away, it's important to store it in the refrigerator. This will slow down the oxidation process and help preserve the flavor and nutrients.

2. Use air-tight containers. To prevent oxidation, store your juices in air-tight containers such as mason jars or glass bottles. Make sure to fill the container all the way to the top so there is no air left in it.

3. Freeze your juices. If you're not going to drink them soon, you can freeze your juices in ice cube trays or other sealed containers. This will keep them fresh for longer periods of time.

4. Use a vacuum sealer. If you plan on storing your juices for long periods of time, a vacuum sealer is a great way to preserve their freshness. When you're ready to drink them, you can thaw them out and enjoy.

5.

Avoid using plastic containers. Plastic containers can leach chemicals into your juices, so it's best to avoid them. Stick with glass jars or bottles for best results.

Juicing is a great way to get your daily dose of fruits and vegetables, and with the right storage techniques, you can make sure your juices stay fresh and delicious. By following these tips, you'll be able to make the most of your juicing experience!

Making Your Juices Taste Better

If you're looking to make your juices taste better, there are several tips and tricks you can use to improve the flavor.

1. Start with the freshest ingredients possible. Fresh fruits and vegetables not only contain more nutrients, but they also have the most intense flavors.

2. Add spices and herbs to your juices to give them an extra flavor boost. A little bit of cinnamon, ginger, or mint can go a long way in enhancing the taste of your juices.

3. Consider adding a few drops of lemon or lime juice to your juices. The acidity in these juices can help to cut through any sweetness and add a nice tangy flavor.

4. Use a variety of fruits and vegetables in your juices. Not only will this give you a wider range of flavors, but it will also add different vitamins and minerals to your juice.

5. Experiment with different combinations of fruits and vegetables. You may be surprised at how different flavors can work together to create a delicious juice.

6. If your juice is too sweet, consider adding a few drops of apple cider vinegar. This will help to balance out the sweetness and add a nice tart flavor.

7. Add a bit of healthy fat to your juices. Adding a tablespoon of nut butter or coconut oil to your juice can help to make it more filling and provide a smooth texture.

8. Use frozen fruits and vegetables in your juices. This will give your juice a thicker texture, and can help to make it more like a smoothie.

9. Use a slow juicer for a smoother texture. Masticating juicers are slower than centrifugal juicers, and can help to create a smoother and more palatable juice.

10. Finally, don't be afraid to experiment! Trying different combinations of ingredients can help you find new and delicious juice recipes.

By following these tips, you can easily make your juices taste better. With a little bit of creativity and experimentation, you can create juices that are packed with flavor and nutrition.

Troubleshooting your Juicer

1. Not enough juice coming out: If you're not getting enough juice out of your juicer, make sure the filter is properly cleaned and that the produce is cut into small enough pieces to fit into the feed chute.

2. Clogged filter: If your filter is clogged, try running some water through the filter to dislodge any debris. If that doesn't work, use a cleaning brush to remove any stuck-on debris.

3. Juicer is noisy: If your juicer is making a lot of noise, make sure all the parts are securely connected and that nothing is

loose. Additionally, check to make sure that all of the produce is cut into small enough pieces to fit into the feed chute.

4. Juicer won't turn on: If your juicer won't turn on, check to make sure it is plugged in and that the power switch is turned on. Additionally, make sure the juicer isn't overloaded with too much produce.

5. Juicer won't turn off: If your juicer won't turn off, make sure the power switch is properly turned off. Additionally, check to make sure the safety switch is properly engaged.

6. Jammed motor: If your motor is jammed, make sure the filter is properly cleaned and that the produce is cut into small enough pieces to fit into the feed chute. Additionally, try using a cleaning brush to remove any stuck-on debris.

7. Overheating motor: If your motor is overheating, make sure the filter is properly cleaned and that the produce is cut into small enough pieces to fit into the feed chute. Additionally, try to avoid overloading the motor with too much produce.

8. Juicer is leaking: If your juicer is leaking, make sure the parts are securely connected and that nothing is loose.

Additionally, check to make sure the filter is properly cleaned and that the produce is cut into small enough pieces to fit into the feed chute.

9. Juicer is vibrating: If your juicer is vibrating, make sure all of the parts are securely connected and that nothing is loose. Additionally, check to make sure the filter is properly cleaned and that the produce is cut into small enough pieces to fit into the feed chute.

10. Juicer is not juicing properly: If your juicer is not juicing properly, make sure the filter is properly cleaned and that the produce is cut into small enough pieces to fit into the feed chute. Additionally, try to avoid overloading the juicer with too much produce.

CHAPTER 3
Common Juicing Problems

1. Pulp Build-up: Pulp build-up is a common problem when juicing and can occur when too much fibre is packed into the juicer. To prevent pulp build-up, make sure to clean the juicer screen and filter regularly. Additionally, you can reduce the amount of fibre in your juice by using a higher ratio of fruits and vegetables with less fibre.

2. Clogging: Clogging is another common problem when juicing. To prevent clogging, make sure to use the proper size of produce for your juicer. If the produce is too large, it can jam up the juicer and cause clogging. Additionally, you can reduce the amount of juice extracted by squeezing the produce gently and not overloading the juicer.

3. Separated Juice: Separated juice occurs when the juice is not mixed properly. To fix this problem, make sure to stir the juice before drinking it and use a juicer that has a mixing function.

4. Foaming: Foaming is caused when too much air is mixed into the juice. To prevent foaming, make sure to use a juicer that has a spinning blade that is designed to reduce the amount of air mixed into the juice. Additionally, you can reduce the amount of air in the juice by allowing the juice to settle before drinking it.

5. Bad Taste: Bad taste is caused by over-extraction, which happens when fruits and vegetables are over-juiced, resulting in a bitter or acidic taste. To prevent this, make sure to use a juicer that has a slow speed setting and reduce the amount of time the produce is being juiced. Additionally, you can reduce the amount of juice extracted by squeezing the produce gently and not overloading the juicer.

6. Skimmed Juice: Skimmed juice is caused by not enough pressure being applied to the produce when juicing. To prevent this, make sure to use a juicer that has a high-powered motor and apply pressure to the produce when juicing. Additionally, you can reduce the amount of juice extracted by squeezing the produce gently and not overloading the juicer.

7. Oxidized Juice: Oxidized juice is caused by oxygen exposure, which can occur when the juice is exposed to air for too long. To reduce oxidation, make sure to drink the juice immediately after juicing and store it in an airtight container. Additionally, you can reduce oxidation by using a juicer that has a vacuum-sealing function.

8. Separated Pulp: Separated pulp is the result of not enough pressure being applied to the produce when juicing. To prevent this, make sure to use a juicer that has a high-powered motor and apply pressure to the produce when juicing. Additionally, you can reduce the amount of juice extracted by squeezing the produce gently and not overloading the juicer.

9. Leaking: Leaking can occur when the juicer is overfilled or not properly assembled. To prevent leaking, make sure to follow the manufacturer's instructions for assembly and use the juicer at the correct capacity. Additionally, you can reduce the amount of juice extracted by squeezing the produce gently and not overloading the juicer.

10. Smells: Smells can occur when the juicer is not cleaned properly or the produce is not fresh. To prevent this, make sure to clean the juicer regularly and use only fresh produce. Additionally, you can reduce the amount of juice extracted by squeezing the produce gently and not overloading the juicer.

How to Avoid Common Mistakes

1. Read the instructions: Be sure to read the instructions that come with your juicer so you know how to properly use and clean your juicer.

2. Prepare the produce: Make sure the fruits and veggies you are juicing are fresh and clean so you have the best tasting juice.

3. Don't overfill: When juicing, it is important to not overfill the juicer as this can cause it to clog.

4. Use the right fruits and vegetables: Not all fruits and vegetables are suitable for juicing, so be sure to choose the right ones.

5. Clean the juicer after each use: Cleaning your juicer after each use will help ensure that it works properly and your juice is as fresh and tasty as possible.

6. Don't add too many ingredients: It is important to not add too many ingredients to your juice as this can make it too sweet or too bitter.

7. Don't leave the juice too long: Juicing takes time and it is important to not leave your juice sitting for too long as this can cause it to spoil.

8. Don't add too much sugar: Adding too much sugar to your juice can cause it to be too sweet and can even affect the health benefits of the juice.

9. Don't add artificial sweeteners: Adding artificial sweeteners to your juice can affect the taste and the health benefits of the juice.

10. Don't over-dilute the juice: Diluting your juice too much can make it too watery and less flavourful.

Juicing for weight Loss

Juicing for weight loss is an effective way to get rid of excess fat and help you reach your ideal weight. It involves replacing meals with freshly-made juices that contain natural and nutrient-packed fruits and vegetables. These nutrient-dense drinks provide the body with vitamins, minerals, and other important nutrients that can help support weight loss.

Juicing for weight loss can be a great way to kick-start a healthier diet and lifestyle. It can help you get rid of unhealthy cravings, reduce overall calorie intake, and provide your body with essential nutrients that can help support a healthy weight loss journey. By replacing meals with freshly-made juices, you can reduce your intake of unhealthy processed foods and instead enjoy a nutrient-dense drink that can help you reach your weight loss goals.

When juicing for weight loss, it's important to choose fruits and vegetables that are low in sugar and high in fibre. This will help ensure that you're getting the most out of your juice and that your body is getting the nutrients it needs to support a healthy weight loss journey. Additionally, it's important to drink plenty of water throughout the day to help keep your body hydrated and to flush out any excess toxins that can slow your progress.

Finally, juicing for weight loss is not a quick fix and it can take some time to see results. However, with dedication and commitment, you can reap the benefits of juicing for weight loss and achieve your desired weight.

CHAPTER 4

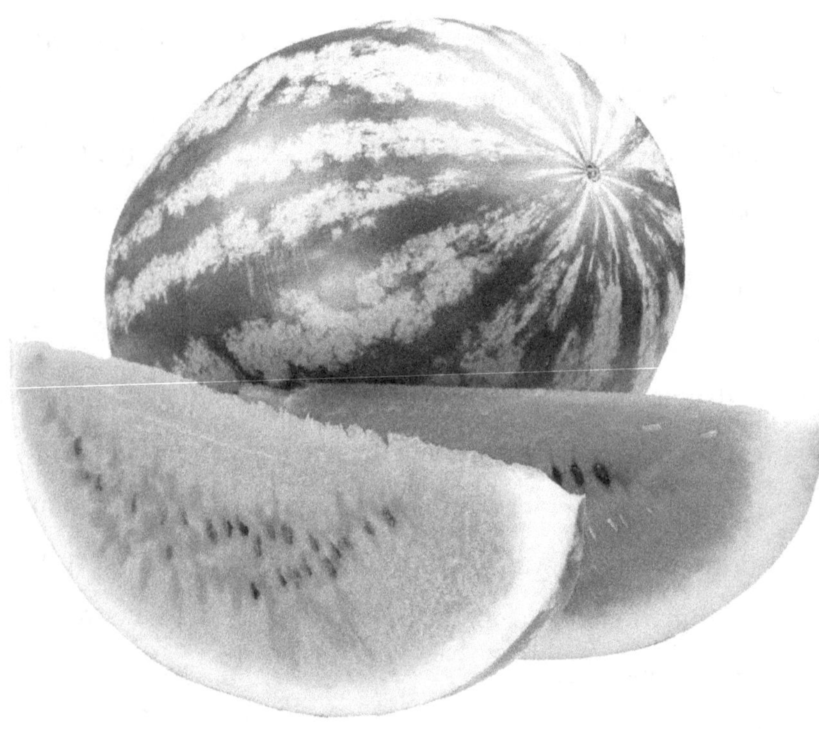

Advanced Juicing Techniques

Advanced juicing techniques involve taking juicing to the next level. These techniques are designed to maximize the benefits of juicing and help you get the most out of your ingredients. Advanced juicing techniques can help you create nutrient-packed juices that are not only delicious but also deliver a number of health benefits.

One of the most popular advanced juicing techniques is juicing with whole fruits and vegetables. Whole juicing involves using the whole fruit or vegetable, including the skin, and juicing it into a smoothie-like beverage. This technique helps to preserve more of the nutrients and enzymes that are naturally found in the produce.

Another advanced juicing technique is green juicing. Green juicing involves using only green vegetables such as kale, spinach, and celery in your juices. This technique helps to create nutrient-packed juices that are rich in vitamins, minerals, and antioxidants. Green juicing can also help to reduce inflammation and boost energy levels.

Finally, one of the most popular advanced juicing techniques is cold-pressed juicing. Cold-pressed juicing involves pressing the ingredients at low temperatures to preserve the maximum amount of nutrients. This technique also helps to create smooth, creamy juices. Cold-pressed juicing can help to boost the nutritional value of your juices and make them more enjoyable to drink.

Advanced juicing techniques can help to create nutrient-packed juices that can help to improve your health and wellness. By incorporating these techniques into your juicing routine, you can get the most out of your ingredients and create delicious, healthy juices.

1. Use a Masticating Juicer: Masticating juicers extract juice from fruits and vegetables by crushing and pressing them, preserving the maximum amount of nutrients from the fruits and vegetables. These types of juicers are great for creating nutrient-rich juices that are packed with vitamins, minerals, and enzymes.

2. Use a High-Speed Blender: High-speed blenders are great for making smoothies and juices that can be consumed immediately, without any additional processing. The blades of a high-speed blender are powerful enough to break down the fibers of fruits and vegetables, allowing you to extract all of the nutrients from them.

3. Use Cold-Pressed Juice: Cold-pressed juices are created by pressing fruits and vegetables at low temperatures and high pressures, preserving the maximum amount of nutrients from the fruits and vegetables. This type of juicing technique is great for creating nutrient-rich juices that are packed with vitamins, minerals, and enzymes.

4. Add Superfoods: Superfoods are nutrient-dense foods that are packed with vitamins, minerals, and antioxidants. Adding superfoods to your juices is a great way to boost the nutritional content of your juices and add additional health benefits.

5. Incorporate Herbs: Adding herbs to your juices is a great way to add flavor as well as additional health benefits. Herbs such as ginger, turmeric, and mint are great for adding flavor and nutrients to your juices.

6. Experiment with Different Ingredients: Experimenting with different fruits, vegetables, and herbs is a great way to create unique and flavorful juices. Trying out different combinations of ingredients can help you find the perfect juice that you enjoy drinking.

BLENDING

Blending involves using high-powered blenders to create nutrient-packed juices. This method is especially effective for those who are looking for a more healthful and nutrient-dense alternative to traditional juicing. With blending, users can benefit from the vitamins and minerals that are released from the whole fruits and vegetables being used, as well as the fiber, which is typically lost in traditional juicing. This type of juicing technique also allows users to make delicious and innovative concoctions that are light and refreshing.

One of the main advantages of Blending is that it preserves the valuable nutrients, vitamins, and minerals that are naturally found in fruits and vegetables. It also helps to retain the fiber content of the fruits and vegetables, which offers additional health benefits. Additionally, this type of juicing technique is extremely versatile, as it allows users to explore a variety of flavor combinations.

To get the most out of Blending, it is important to use high-powered blenders. This type of blender is necessary to break down the tough fibers of the fruits and vegetables, which is essential for unlocking the maximum amount of nutrients. It is also important to use fresh, ripe fruits and vegetables for the best results. Additionally, it is important to use cold-pressed juices in order to preserve the important nutrients and vitamins.

Blending is a great way to get more nutrients, vitamins, and minerals from fruits and vegetables. It is also a great way to explore different flavor combinations and create delicious and nutritious drinks. With the right equipment and ingredients, this type of juicing technique can be a great addition to any health-conscious lifestyle.

INFUSING

Infusing combines the power of fresh juices with the benefits of essential oils. This technique allows you to enjoy the taste of fresh juices while getting the benefits of essential oils, without the overwhelming aroma or taste of the oil. Essential oils are extremely concentrated and potent, and infusing them into juice can be a great way to reap their benefits without having to consume them directly.

The process of advanced juicing technique infusing involves adding a few drops of your favorite essential oil to a glass or bottle of freshly-made juice. You can choose from a variety of essential oils, depending on the therapeutic benefits you're looking for. For example, lavender essential oil promotes relaxation and reduces stress, while peppermint oil aids digestion and can help alleviate nausea.

Once you've chosen your oil, add a few drops to the juice and give it a gentle stir. You can also add a few drops of the oil to a bottle of pre-made juice if you're in a pinch. The essential oil should be completely dispersed throughout the juice before you drink it.

When choosing an essential oil to infuse into your juice, make sure to select one that is safe for ingestion. Some essential oils can be harmful if ingested, so be sure to research the oil you're using before consuming it.

Advanced juicing technique infusing is a great way to get the benefits of essential oils without having to consume them directly. It's also an easy way to add flavor and nutrition to your favorite beverages. With a little bit of research and experimentation, you can find the perfect combination of essential oil and juice to create a delicious, healthful drink.

CHAPTER 5

Recipes

Fruit Juices
Strawberry Banana Juice

Ingredients: 2 fresh strawberries, 1 banana, 1 cup of ice, 2 tablespoons of honey, 1 cup of orange juice

Steps:

1. Peel the banana and cut it into small pieces.

2. Wash and hull the strawberries.

3. Place the banana, strawberries, honey, orange juice, and ice in a blender.

4. Blend the ingredients until smooth.

5. Serve the juice immediately.

Blueberry Pineapple Juice

Ingredients: 1 cup fresh blueberries, 1 cup fresh pineapple, 1 cup of ice, 2 tablespoons of honey, 1 cup of orange juice

Steps:

1. Peel and chop the pineapple into small pieces.

2. Wash and hull the blueberries.

3. Place the pineapple, blueberries, honey, orange juice, and ice in a blender.

4. Blend the ingredients until smooth.

5. Serve the juice immediately.

Watermelon Coconut Juice

Ingredients: 2 cups of fresh watermelon cubes, 1/2 cup of coconut milk, 1 cup of ice, 2 tablespoons of honey

Steps:

1. Peel and cube the watermelon.

2. Place the watermelon cubes, coconut milk, honey, and ice in a blender.

3. Blend the ingredients until smooth.

4. Serve the juice immediately.

Apple Carrot Juice

Ingredients: 2 apples, 2 carrots, 1 cup of ice, 2 tablespoons of honey, 1 cup of orange juice

Steps:

1. Peel and chop the apples and carrots into small pieces.

2. Place the apples, carrots, honey, orange juice, and ice in a blender.

3. Blend the ingredients until smooth.

4. Serve the juice immediately.

Mango Peach Juice

Ingredients: 2 mangos, 2 peaches, 1 cup of ice, 2 tablespoons of honey, 1 cup of orange juice

Steps:

1. Peel and chop the mangos and peaches into small pieces.

2. Place the mangos, peaches, honey, orange juice, and ice in a blender.

3. Blend the ingredients until smooth.

4. Serve the juice immediately.

Raspberry Banana Juice

Ingredients: 2 cups of fresh raspberries, 1 banana, 1 cup of ice, 2 tablespoons of honey, 1 cup of orange juice

Steps:

1. Peel the banana and cut it into small pieces.

2. Wash and hull the raspberries.

3. Place the banana, raspberries, honey, orange juice, and ice in a blender.

4. Blend the ingredients until smooth.

5. Serve the juice immediately.

Papaya Orange Juice

Ingredients: 2 papayas, 3 oranges, 1 cup of ice, 2 tablespoons of honey

Steps:

1. Peel and chop the papayas and oranges into small pieces.

2. Place the papayas, oranges, honey, and ice in a blender.

3. Blend the ingredients until smooth.

4. Serve the juice immediately.

Pineapple Coconut Juice

Ingredients: 1 cup fresh pineapple, 1/2 cup of coconut milk, 1 cup of ice, 2 tablespoons of honey

Steps:

1. Peel and chop the pineapple into small pieces.

2. Place the pineapple, coconut milk, honey, and ice in a blender.

3. Blend the ingredients until smooth.

4. Serve the juice immediately.

Pear Kiwi Juice

Ingredients: 2 pears, 2 kiwis, 1 cup of ice, 2 tablespoons of honey, 1 cup of orange juice

Steps:

1. Peel and chop the pears and kiwis into small pieces.

2. Place the pears, kiwis, honey, orange juice, and ice in a blender.

3. Blend the ingredients until smooth.

4. Serve the juice immediately.

Cherry Plum Juice

Ingredients: 2 cups of fresh cherries, 1 plum, 1 cup of ice, 2 tablespoons of honey, 1 cup of orange juice

Steps:

1. Pit and hull the cherries.

2. Peel and chop the plum into small pieces.

3. Place the cherries, plum, honey, orange juice, and ice in a blender.

4. Blend the ingredients until smooth.

5. Serve the juice immediately.

Avocado Pear Juice

Ingredients: 1 avocado, 2 pears, 1 cup of ice, 2 tablespoons of honey, 1 cup of orange juice

Steps:

1. Peel and pit the avocado.

2. Peel and chop the pears into small pieces.

3. Place the avocado, pears, honey, orange juice, and ice in a blender.

4. Blend the ingredients until smooth.

5. Serve the juice immediately.

Apple Peach Juice

Ingredients: 2 apples, 2 peaches, 1 cup of ice, 2 tablespoons of honey, 1 cup of orange juice

Steps:

1. Peel and chop the apples and peaches into small pieces.

2. Place the apples, peaches, honey, orange juice, and ice in a blender.

3. Blend the ingredients until smooth.

4. Serve the juice immediately.

Mango Coconut Juice

Ingredients: 2 mangos, 1/2 cup of coconut milk, 1 cup of ice, 2 tablespoons of honey

Steps:

1. Peel and chop the mangos into small pieces.

2. Place the mangos, coconut milk, honey, and ice in a blender.

3. Blend the ingredients until smooth.

4. Serve the juice immediately.

Strawberry Apple Juice

Ingredients: 2 fresh strawberries, 2 apples, 1 cup of ice, 2 tablespoons of honey, 1 cup of orange juice

Steps:

1. Peel and chop the apples into small pieces.

2. Wash and hull the strawberries.

3. Place the apples, strawberries, honey, orange juice, and ice in a blender.

4. Blend the ingredients until smooth.

5. Serve the juice immediately.

Pineapple Banana Juice

Ingredients: 1 cup fresh pineapple, 1 banana, 1 cup of ice, 2 tablespoons of honey, 1 cup of orange juice

Steps:

1. Peel and chop the pineapple and banana into small pieces.

2. Place the pineapple, banana, honey, orange juice, and ice in a blender.

3. Blend the ingredients until smooth.

4. Serve the juice immediately.

Watermelon Pear Juice

Ingredients: 2 cups of fresh watermelon cubes, 2 pears, 1 cup of ice, 2 tablespoons of honey

Steps:

1. Peel and cube the watermelon.

2. Peel and chop the pears into small pieces.

3. Place the watermelon cubes, pears, honey, and ice in a blender.

4. Blend the ingredients until smooth.

5. Serve the juice immediately.

Cherry Apple Juice

Ingredients: 2 cups of fresh cherries, 2 apples, 1 cup of ice, 2 tablespoons of honey, 1 cup of orange juice

Steps:

1. Pit and hull the cherries.

2. Peel and chop the apples into small pieces.

3. Place the cherries, apples, honey, orange juice, and ice in a blender.

4. Blend the ingredients until smooth.

5. Serve the juice immediately.

Papaya Banana Juice

Ingredients: 2 papayas, 1 banana, 1 cup of ice, 2 tablespoons of honey, 1 cup of orange juice

Steps:

1. Peel and chop the papayas and banana into small pieces.

2. Place the papayas, banana, honey, orange juice, and ice in a blender.

3. Blend the ingredients until smooth.

4. Serve the juice immediately.

Mango Carrot Juice

Ingredients: 2 mangos, 2 carrots, 1 cup of ice, 2 tablespoons of honey, 1 cup of orange juice

Steps:

1. Peel and chop the mangos and carrots into small pieces.

2. Place the mangos, carrots, honey, orange juice, and ice in a blender.

3. Blend the ingredients until smooth.

4. Serve the juice immediately.

Blueberry Banana Juice

Ingredients: 1 cup fresh blueberries, 1 banana, 1 cup of ice, 2 tablespoons of honey, 1 cup of orange juice

Steps:

1. Peel and chop the banana into small pieces.

2. Wash and hull the blueberries.

3. Place the banana, blueberries, honey, orange juice, and ice in a blender.

4. Blend the ingredients until smooth.

5. Serve the juice immediately.

Pineapple Papaya Juice

Ingredients: 1 cup fresh pineapple, 2 papayas, 1 cup of ice, 2 tablespoons of honey

Steps:

1. Peel and chop the pineapple and papayas into small pieces.

2. Place the pineapple, papayas, honey, and ice in a blender.

3. Blend the ingredients until smooth.

4. Serve the juice immediately.

Avocado Mango Juice

Ingredients: 1 avocado, 2 mangos, 1 cup of ice, 2 tablespoons of honey, 1 cup of orange juice

Steps:

1. Peel and pit the avocado.

2. Peel and chop the mangos into small pieces.

3. Place the avocado, mangos, honey, orange juice, and ice in a blender.

4. Blend the ingredients until smooth.

5. Serve the juice immediately.

Raspberry Coconut Juice

Ingredients: 2 cups of fresh raspberries, 1/2 cup of coconut milk, 1 cup of ice, 2 tablespoons of honey

Steps:

1. Wash and hull the raspberries.

2. Place the raspberries, coconut milk, honey, and ice in a blender.

3. Blend the ingredients until smooth.

4. Serve the juice immediately.

Kiwi Pear Juice

Ingredients: 2 kiwis, 2 pears, 1 cup of ice, 2 tablespoons of honey, 1 cup of orange juice

Steps:

1. Peel and chop the kiwis and pears into small pieces.

2. Place the kiwis, pears, honey, orange juice, and ice in a blender.

3. Blend the ingredients until smooth.

4. Serve the juice immediately.

Apple Kiwi Juice

Ingredients: 2 apples, 2 kiwis, 1 cup of ice, 2 tablespoons of honey, 1 cup of orange juice

Steps:

1. Peel and chop the apples and kiwis into small pieces.

2. Place the apples, kiwis, honey, orange juice, and ice in a blender.

3. Blend the ingredients until smooth.

4. Serve the juice immediately.

Cherry Plum Juice

Ingredients: 2 cups of fresh cherries, 1 plum, 1 cup of ice, 2 tablespoons of honey, 1 cup of orange juice

Steps:

1. Pit and hull the cherries.

2. Peel and chop the plum into small pieces.

3. Place the cherries, plum, honey, orange juice, and ice in a blender.

4. Blend the ingredients until smooth.

5. Serve the juice immediately.

Peach Coconut Juice

Ingredients: 2 peaches, 1/2 cup of coconut milk, 1 cup of ice, 2 tablespoons of honey

Steps:

1. Peel and chop the peaches into small pieces.

2. Place the peaches, coconut milk, honey, and ice in a blender.

3. Blend the ingredients until smooth.

4. Serve the juice immediately.

Pear Orange Juice

Ingredients: 2 pears, 3 oranges, 1 cup of ice, 2 tablespoons of honey

Steps:

1. Peel and chop the pears and oranges into small pieces.

2. Place the pears, oranges, honey, and ice in a blender.

3. Blend the ingredients until smooth.

4. Serve the juice immediately.

Watermelon Apple Juice

Ingredients: 2 cups of fresh watermelon cubes, 2 apples, 1 cup of ice, 2 tablespoons of honey, 1 cup of orange juice

Steps:

1. Peel and cube the watermelon.

2. Peel and chop the apples into small pieces.

3. Place the watermelon cubes, apples, honey, orange juice, and ice in a blender.

4. Blend the ingredients until smooth.

5. Serve the juice immediately.

Papaya Pineapple Juice

Ingredients: 2 papayas, 1 cup fresh pineapple, 1 cup of ice, 2 tablespoons of honey

Steps:

1. Peel and chop the papayas and pineapple into small pieces.

2. Place the papayas, pineapple, honey, and ice in a blender.

3. Blend the ingredients until smooth.

4. Serve the juice immediately.

Raspberry Banana Juice

Ingredients: 2 cups of fresh raspberries, 1 banana, 1 cup of ice, 2 tablespoons of honey, 1 cup of orange juice

Steps:

1. Peel and chop the banana into small pieces.

2. Wash and hull the raspberries.

3. Place the banana, raspberries, honey, orange juice, and ice in a blender.

4. Blend the ingredients until smooth.

5. Serve the juice immediately.

Blueberry Coconut Juice

Ingredients: 1 cup fresh blueberries, 1/2 cup of coconut milk, 1 cup of ice, 2 tablespoons of honey

Steps:

1. Wash and hull the blueberries.

2. Place the blueberries, coconut milk, honey, and ice in a blender.

3. Blend the ingredients until smooth.

4. Serve the juice immediately.

CHAPTER 6
Vegetable Based Juices

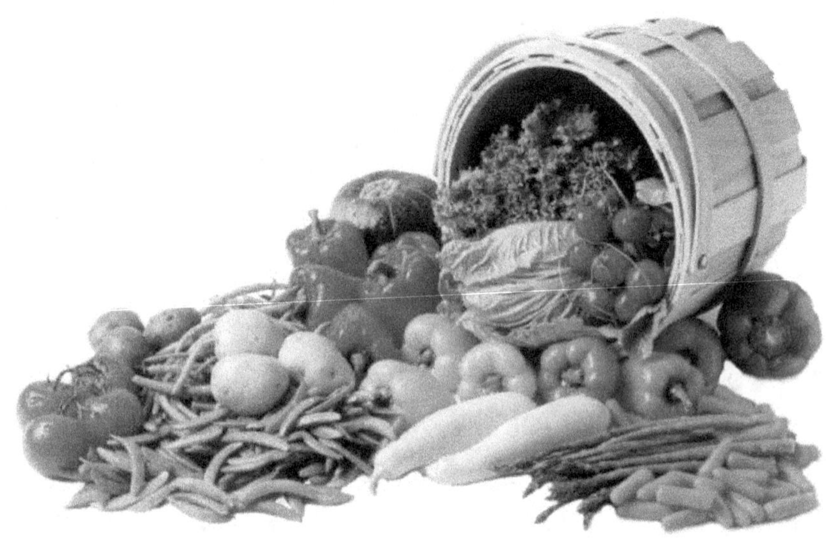

Carrot Apple Juice

Ingredients: 2 apples, 4 carrots, 1 cup of water

Steps:

1. Peel and cut the apples and carrots into small pieces.

2. Place the apple and carrot pieces into a blender.

3. Add a cup of water.

4. Blend until smooth.

5. Strain the juice and serve.

Beetroot Spinach Juice

Ingredients: 2 beets, 1 cup of spinach, 1 cup of water

Steps:

1. Peel and cut the beets into small pieces.

2. Place the beet pieces into a blender.

3. Add a cup of spinach and a cup of water.

4. Blend until smooth.

5. Strain the juice and serve.

Cucumber Celery Juice

Ingredients: 1 cucumber, 2 stalks of celery, 1 cup of water

Steps:

1. Peel and cut the cucumber into small pieces.

2. Chop the celery into small pieces.

3. Place the cucumber and celery pieces into a blender.

4. Add a cup of water.

5. Blend until smooth.

6. Strain the juice and serve.

Kale Tomato Juice

Ingredients: 1 cup of kale, 2 tomatoes, 1 cup of water

Steps:

1. Chop the kale and tomatoes into small pieces.

2. Place the kale and tomato pieces into a blender.

3. Add a cup of water.

4. Blend until smooth.

5. Strain the juice and serve.

Broccoli Pear Juice

Ingredients: 1 head of broccoli, 2 pears, 1 cup of water

Steps:

1. Cut the broccoli into small pieces.

2. Peel and cut the pears into small pieces.

3. Place the broccoli and pear pieces into a blender.

4. Add a cup of water.

5. Blend until smooth.

6. Strain the juice and serve.

Zucchini Carrot Juice

Ingredients: 1 zucchini, 2 carrots, 1 cup of water

Steps:

1. Peel and cut the zucchini and carrots into small pieces.

2. Place the zucchini and carrot pieces into a blender.

3. Add a cup of water.

4. Blend until smooth.

5. Strain the juice and serve.

Cauliflower Apple Juice

Ingredients: 1 head of cauliflower, 2 apples, 1 cup of water

Steps:

1. Break the cauliflower into small florets.

2. Peel and cut the apples into small pieces.

3. Place the cauliflower and apple pieces into a blender.

4. Add a cup of water.

5. Blend until smooth.

6. Strain the juice and serve.

Sweet Potato Orange Juice

Ingredients: 1 sweet potato, 2 oranges, 1 cup of water

Steps:

1. Peel and cut the sweet potato into small pieces.

2. Peel and cut the oranges into small pieces.

3. Place the sweet potato and orange pieces into a blender.

4. Add a cup of water.

5. Blend until smooth.

6. Strain the juice and serve.

Squash Pineapple Juice

Ingredients: 1 squash, 1/2 pineapple, 1 cup of water

Steps:

1. Peel and cut the squash into small pieces.

2. Peel and cut the pineapple into small pieces.

3. Place the squash and pineapple pieces into a blender.

4. Add a cup of water.

5. Blend until smooth.

6. Strain the juice and serve.

Radish Pear Juice

Ingredients: 5 radishes, 2 pears, 1 cup of water

Steps:

1. Peel and cut the radishes into small pieces.

2. Peel and cut the pears into small pieces.

3. Place the radish and pear pieces into a blender.

4. Add a cup of water.

5. Blend until smooth.

6. Strain the juice and serve.

Asparagus Lemon Juice

Ingredients: 1 bundle of asparagus, 2 lemons, 1 cup of water

Steps:

1. Cut the asparagus into small pieces.

2. Peel and cut the lemons into small pieces.

3. Place the asparagus and lemon pieces into a blender.

4. Add a cup of water.

5. Blend until smooth.

6. Strain the juice and serve.

Potato Grape Juice

Ingredients: 1 potato, 1 cup of grapes, 1 cup of water

Steps:

1. Peel and cut the potato into small pieces.

2. Place the potato pieces into a blender.

3. Add a cup of grapes and a cup of water.

4. Blend until smooth.

5. Strain the juice and serve.

Bell Pepper Watermelon Juice

Ingredients: 1 bell pepper, 1/2 watermelon, 1 cup of water

Steps:

1. Cut the bell pepper into small pieces.

2. Peel and cut the watermelon into small pieces.

3. Place the bell pepper and watermelon pieces into a blender.

4. Add a cup of water.

5. Blend until smooth.

6. Strain the juice and serve.

Eggplant Grapefruit Juice

Ingredients: 1 eggplant, 1 grapefruit, 1 cup of water

Steps:

1. Peel and cut the eggplant into small pieces.

2. Peel and cut the grapefruit into small pieces.

3. Place the eggplant and grapefruit pieces into a blender.

4. Add a cup of water.

5. Blend until smooth.

6. Strain the juice and serve.

Leek Strawberry Juice

Ingredients: 2 leeks, 1 cup of strawberries, 1 cup of water

Steps:

1. Cut the leeks into small pieces.

2. Place the leek pieces into a blender.

3. Add a cup of strawberries and a cup of water.

4. Blend until smooth.

5. Strain the juice and serve.

Fennel Cucumber Juice

Ingredients: 2 fennel bulbs, 1 cucumber, 1 cup of water

Steps:

1. Cut the fennel bulbs into small pieces.

2. Peel and cut the cucumber into small pieces.

3. Place the fennel and cucumber pieces into a blender.

4. Add a cup of water.

5. Blend until smooth.

6. Strain the juice and serve.

Mushroom Avocado Juice

Ingredients: 1 cup of mushrooms, 1 avocado, 1 cup of water

Steps:

1. Cut the mushrooms into small pieces.

2. Peel and cut the avocado into small pieces.

3. Place the mushroom and avocado pieces into a blender.

4. Add a cup of water.

5. Blend until smooth.

6. Strain the juice and serve.

Artichoke Apple Juice

Ingredients: 2 artichokes, 2 apples, 1 cup of water

Steps:

1. Peel and cut the artichokes into small pieces.

2. Peel and cut the apples into small pieces.

3. Place the artichoke and apple pieces into a blender.

4. Add a cup of water.

5. Blend until smooth.

6. Strain the juice and serve.

Parsnip Mango Juice

Ingredients: 3 parsnips, 1 mango, 1 cup of water

Steps:

1. Peel and cut the parsnips into small pieces.

2. Peel and cut the mango into small pieces.

3. Place the parsnip and mango pieces into a blender.

4. Add a cup of water.

5. Blend until smooth.

6. Strain the juice and serve.

Rutabaga Blueberry Juice

Ingredients: 1 rutabaga, 1 cup of blueberries, 1 cup of water

Steps:

1. Peel and cut the rutabaga into small pieces.

2. Place the rutabaga pieces into a blender.

3. Add a cup of blueberries and a cup of water.

4. Blend until smooth.

5. Strain the juice and serve.

Turnip Peach Juice

Ingredients: 2 turnips, 2 peaches, 1 cup of water

Steps:

1. Peel and cut the turnips into small pieces.

2. Peel and cut the peaches into small pieces.

3. Place the turnip and peach pieces into a blender.

4. Add a cup of water.

5. Blend until smooth.

6. Strain the juice and serve.

Swiss Chard Orange Juice

Ingredients: 1 bunch of swiss chard, 2 oranges, 1 cup of water

Steps:

1. Cut the swiss chard into small pieces.

2. Peel and cut the oranges into small pieces.

3. Place the swiss chard and orange pieces into a blender.

4. Add a cup of water.

5. Blend until smooth.

6. Strain the juice and serve.

Bok Choy Pineapple Juice

Ingredients: 1 head of bok choy, 1/2 pineapple, 1 cup of water

Steps:

1. Cut the bok choy into small pieces.

2. Peel and cut the pineapple into small pieces.

3. Place the bok choy and pineapple pieces into a blender.

4. Add a cup of water.

5. Blend until smooth.

6. Strain the juice and serve.

Mustard Greens Banana Juice

Ingredients: 1 bunch of mustard greens, 1 banana, 1 cup of water

Steps:

1. Cut the mustard greens into small pieces.

2. Peel and cut the banana into small pieces.

3. Place the mustard greens and banana pieces into a blender.

4. Add a cup of water.

5. Blend until smooth.

6. Strain the juice and serve.

Pumpkin Apple Juice

Ingredients: 1/2 pumpkin, 2 apples, 1 cup of water

Steps:

1. Peel and cut the pumpkin into small pieces.

2. Peel and cut the apples into small pieces.

3. Place the pumpkin and apple pieces into a blender.

4. Add a cup of water.

5. Blend until smooth.

6. Strain the juice and serve.

Butternut Squash Pear Juice

Ingredients: 1/2 butternut squash, 2 pears, 1 cup of water

Steps:

1. Peel and cut the butternut squash into small pieces.

2. Peel and cut the pears into small pieces.

3. Place the butternut squash and pear pieces into a blender.

4. Add a cup of water.

5. Blend until smooth.

6. Strain the juice and serve.

Tomato Apricot Juice

Ingredients: 2 tomatoes, 2 apricots, 1 cup of water

Steps:

1. Cut the tomatoes into small pieces.

2. Peel and cut the apricots into small pieces.

3. Place the tomato and apricot pieces into a blender.

4. Add a cup of water.

5. Blend until smooth.

6. Strain the juice and serve.

Sweet Pepper Grape Juice

Ingredients: 2 sweet peppers, 1 cup of grapes, 1 cup of water

Steps:

1. Cut the sweet peppers into small pieces.

2. Place the sweet pepper pieces into a blender.

3. Add a cup of grapes and a cup of water.

4. Blend until smooth.

5. Strain the juice and serve.

Celery Kiwi Juice

Ingredients: 2 stalks of celery, 2 kiwis, 1 cup of water

Steps:

1. Chop the celery into small pieces.

2. Peel and cut the kiwis into small pieces.

3. Place the celery and kiwi pieces into a blender.

4. Add a cup of water.

5. Blend until smooth.

6. Strain the juice and serve.

Garlic Grape Juice

Ingredients: 10 cloves of garlic, 1 cup of grapes, 1 cup of water

Steps:

1. Peel and chop the garlic into small pieces.

2. Place the garlic pieces into a blender.

3. Add a cup of grapes and a cup of water.

4. Blend until smooth.

5. Strain the juice and serve.

Endive Papaya Juice

Ingredients: 2 endives, 1 papaya, 1 cup of water

Steps:

1. Cut the endives into small pieces.

2. Peel and cut the papaya into small pieces.

3. Place the endive and papaya pieces into a blender.

4. Add a cup of water.

5. Blend until smooth.

6. Strain the juice and serve.

Radicchio Banana Juice

Ingredients: 1 head of radicchio, 1 banana, 1 cup of water

Steps:

1. Cut the radicchio into small pieces.

2. Peel and cut the banana into small pieces.

3. Place the radicchio and banana pieces into a blender.

4. Add a cup of water.

5. Blend until smooth.

6. Strain the juice and serve.

CHAPTER 7

Green Juices

Green Mango Juice

Ingredients: 1 cup mango cubes, 1 cup fresh spinach leaves, 2 teaspoons honey, 1/2 cup water

Steps:

1. Add mango cubes, fresh spinach leaves and honey to a blender.

2. Blend until smooth.

3. Add water and blend again until desired consistency is achieved.

4. Serve chilled.

Apple Spinach Juice

Ingredients: 1 green apple, 1 cup fresh spinach leaves, 1 teaspoon honey, 1/2 cup water

Steps:

1. Peel and core the apple and cut into cubes.

2. Add the apple cubes, fresh spinach leaves and honey to a blender.

3. Blend until smooth.

4. Add water and blend again until desired consistency is achieved.

5. Serve chilled.

Green Coconut Juice

Ingredients: 1/2 cup coconut milk, 1 cup fresh spinach leaves, 2 teaspoons honey, 1/2 cup water

Steps:

1. Add coconut milk, fresh spinach leaves and honey to a blender.

2. Blend until smooth.

3. Add water and blend again until desired consistency is achieved.

4. Serve chilled.

Celery Cucumber Juice

Ingredients: 1 stalk celery, 1/2 cucumber, 1/2 cup fresh parsley leaves, 1 teaspoon honey, 1/2 cup water

Steps:

1. Peel and cut the cucumber into small pieces.

2. Add the celery, cucumber, parsley leaves and honey to a blender.

3. Blend until smooth.

4. Add water and blend again until desired consistency is achieved.

5. Serve chilled.

Broccoli Kale Juice

Ingredients: 1/2 cup broccoli florets, 1/2 cup kale leaves, 1 teaspoon honey, 1/2 cup water

Steps:

1. Add the broccoli florets, kale leaves and honey to a blender.

2. Blend until smooth.

3. Add water and blend again until desired consistency is achieved.

4. Serve chilled.

Green Banana Juice

Ingredients: 1 ripe banana, 1 cup fresh spinach leaves, 2 teaspoons honey, 1/2 cup water

Steps:

1. Peel the banana and cut it into cubes.

2. Add the banana cubes, fresh spinach leaves and honey to a blender.

3. Blend until smooth.

4. Add water and blend again until desired consistency is achieved.

5. Serve chilled.

Green Avocado Juice

Ingredients: 1/2 avocado, 1 cup fresh spinach leaves, 2 teaspoons honey, 1/2 cup water

Steps:

1. Peel and cut the avocado into cubes.

2. Add the avocado cubes, fresh spinach leaves and honey to a blender.

3. Blend until smooth.

4. Add water and blend again until desired consistency is achieved.

5. Serve chilled.

Pineapple Spinach Juice

Ingredients: 1 cup pineapple cubes, 1 cup fresh spinach leaves, 2 teaspoons honey, 1/2 cup water

Steps:

1. Add pineapple cubes, fresh spinach leaves and honey to a blender.

2. Blend until smooth.

3. Add water and blend again until desired consistency is achieved.

4. Serve chilled.

Green Grape Juice

Ingredients: 1 cup green grapes, 1 cup fresh spinach leaves, 2 teaspoons honey, 1/2 cup water

Steps:

1. Add green grapes, fresh spinach leaves and honey to a blender.

2. Blend until smooth.

3. Add water and blend again until desired consistency is achieved.

4. Serve chilled.

Green Lemonade

Ingredients: 1/2 cup freshly squeezed lemon juice, 1 cup fresh spinach leaves, 2 teaspoons honey, 1/2 cup water

Steps:

1. Add freshly squeezed lemon juice, fresh spinach leaves and honey to a blender.

2. Blend until smooth.

3. Add water and blend again until desired consistency is achieved.

4. Serve chilled.

Carrot Spinach Juice

Ingredients: 1 large carrot, 1 cup fresh spinach leaves, 2 teaspoons honey, 1/2 cup water

Steps:

1. Peel and cut the carrot into cubes.

2. Add the carrot cubes, fresh spinach leaves and honey to a blender.

3. Blend until smooth.

4. Add water and blend again until desired consistency is achieved.

5. Serve chilled.

Green Orange Juice

Ingredients: 1 large orange, 1 cup fresh spinach leaves, 2 teaspoons honey, 1/2 cup water

Steps:

1. Peel and cut the orange into small bits.

2. Add the orange cubes, fresh spinach leaves and honey to a blender.

3. Blend until smooth.

4. Add water and blend again until desired consistency is achieved.

5. Serve chilled.

Green Papaya Juice

Ingredients: 1/2 cup papaya cubes, 1 cup fresh spinach leaves, 2 teaspoons honey, 1/2 cup water

Steps:

1. Add papaya cubes, fresh spinach leaves and honey to a blender.

2. Blend until smooth.

3. Add water and blend again until desired consistency is achieved.

4. Serve chilled.

Green Peach Juice

Ingredients: 1 large peach, 1 cup fresh spinach leaves, 2 teaspoons honey, 1/2 cup water

Steps:

1. Peel and cut the peach into small pieces.

2. Add the peach cubes, fresh spinach leaves and honey to a blender.

3. Blend until smooth.

4. Add water and blend again until desired consistency is achieved.

5. Serve chilled.

Cucumber Apple Juice

Ingredients: 1/2 cucumber, 1 green apple, 1 teaspoon honey, 1/2 cup water

Steps:

1. Peel and core the apple and cut into small pieces.

2. Peel and cut the cucumber into cubes.

3. Add the apple cubes, cucumber cubes and honey to a blender.

4. Blend until smooth.

5. Add water and blend again until desired consistency is achieved.

6. Serve chilled.

Cilantro Spinach Juice

Ingredients: 1/2 cup fresh cilantro leaves, 1 cup fresh spinach leaves, 2 teaspoons honey, 1/2 cup water

Steps:

1. Add the cilantro leaves, fresh spinach leaves and honey to a blender.

2. Blend until smooth.

3. Add water and blend again until desired consistency is achieved.

4. Serve chilled.

Green Melon Juice

Ingredients: 1/2 cup cubed honeydew melon, 1 cup fresh spinach leaves, 2 teaspoons honey, 1/2 cup water

Steps:

1. Add honeydew melon cubes, fresh spinach leaves and honey to a blender.

2. Blend until smooth.

3. Add water and blend again until desired consistency is achieved.

4. Serve chilled.

Green Grapefruit Juice

Ingredients: 1/2 cup freshly squeezed grapefruit juice, 1 cup fresh spinach leaves, 2 teaspoons honey, 1/2 cup water

Steps:

1. Add freshly squeezed grapefruit juice, fresh spinach leaves and honey to a blender.

2. Blend until smooth.

3. Add water and blend again until desired consistency is achieved.

4. Serve chilled.

Cucumber Celery Juice

Ingredients: 1/2 cucumber, 1 stalk celery, 1 teaspoon honey, 1/2 cup water

Steps:

1. Peel and cut the cucumber into cubes.

2. Add the cucumber cubes, celery and honey to a blender.

3. Blend until smooth.

4. Add water and blend again until desired consistency is achieved.

5. Serve chilled.

Green Smoothie

Ingredients: 1 cup frozen banana slices, 1 cup fresh spinach leaves, 2 teaspoons honey, 1/2 cup water

Steps:

1. Add frozen banana slices, fresh spinach leaves and honey to a blender.

2. Blend until smooth.

3. Add water and blend again until desired consistency is achieved.

4. Serve chilled.

Green Pineapple Juice

Ingredients: 1 cup pineapple cubes, 1 cup fresh spinach leaves, 2 teaspoons honey, 1/2 cup water

Steps:

1. Add pineapple cubes, fresh spinach leaves and honey to a blender.

2. Blend until smooth.

3. Add water and blend again until desired consistency is achieved.

4. Serve chilled.

Beet Spinach Juice

Ingredients: 1/2 cup cooked beet cubes, 1 cup fresh spinach leaves, 2 teaspoons honey, 1/2 cup water

Steps:

1. Add cooked beet cubes, fresh spinach leaves and honey to a blender.

2. Blend until smooth.

3. Add water and blend again until desired consistency is achieved.

4. Serve chilled.

Green Melon Mint Juice

Ingredients: 1/2 cup cubed honeydew melon, 1/2 cup fresh mint leaves, 1 teaspoon honey, 1/2 cup water

Steps:

1. Add honeydew melon cubes, fresh mint leaves and honey to a blender.

2. Blend until smooth.

3. Add water and blend again until desired consistency is achieved.

4. Serve chilled.

Green Apple Juice

Ingredients: 1 green apple, 1 cup fresh spinach leaves, 2 teaspoons honey, 1/2 cup water

Steps:

1. Peel and core the apple and cut into small pieces.

2. Add the apple cubes, fresh spinach leaves and honey to a blender.

3. Blend until smooth.

4. Add water and blend again until desired consistency is achieved.

5. Serve chilled.

Green Berry Juice

Ingredients: 1/2 cup blueberries, 1/2 cup raspberries, 1 cup fresh spinach leaves, 2 teaspoons honey, 1/2 cup water

Steps:

1. Add blueberries, raspberries, fresh spinach leaves and honey to a blender.

2. Blend until smooth.

3. Add water and blend again until desired consistency is achieved.

4. Serve chilled.

Avocado Spinach Juice

Ingredients: 1/2 avocado, 1 cup fresh spinach leaves, 2 teaspoons honey, 1/2 cup water

Steps:

1. Peel and cut the avocado into small pieces.

2. Add the avocado cubes, fresh spinach leaves and honey to a blender.

3. Blend until smooth.

4. Add water and blend again until desired consistency is achieved.

5. Serve chilled.

Cucumber Dill Juice

Ingredients: 1/2 cucumber, 1/2 cup fresh dill leaves, 1 teaspoon honey, 1/2 cup water

Steps:

1. Peel and cut the cucumber into small pieces.

2. Add the cucumber cubes, fresh dill leaves and honey to a blender.

3. Blend until smooth.

4. Add water and blend again until desired consistency is achieved.

5. Serve chilled.

Green Tomato Juice

Ingredients: 1/2 cup tomato cubes, 1 cup fresh spinach leaves, 2 teaspoons honey, 1/2 cup water

Steps:

1. Add tomato cubes, fresh spinach leaves and honey to a blender.

2. Blend until smooth.

3. Add water and blend again until desired consistency is achieved.

4. Serve chilled.

Green Mango Pineapple Juice

Ingredients: 1 cup mango cubes, 1 cup pineapple cubes, 1 cup fresh spinach leaves, 2 teaspoons honey, 1/2 cup water

Steps:

1. Add mango cubes, pineapple cubes, fresh spinach leaves and honey to a blender.

2. Blend until smooth.

3. Add water and blend again until desired consistency is achieved.

4. Serve chilled.

Green Lemon Mint Juice

Ingredients: 1/2 cup freshly squeezed lemon juice, 1/2 cup fresh mint leaves, 1 teaspoon honey, 1/2 cup water

Steps:

1. Add freshly squeezed lemon juice, fresh mint leaves and honey to a blender.

2. Blend until smooth.

3. Add water and blend again until desired consistency is achieved.

4. Serve chilled.

Cucumber Parsley Juice

Ingredients: 1/2 cucumber, 1/2 cup fresh parsley leaves, 1 teaspoon honey, 1/2 cup water

Steps:

1. Peel and cut the cucumber into small pieces.

2. Add the cucumber cubes, fresh parsley leaves and honey to a blender.

3. Blend until smooth.

4. Add water and blend again until desired consistency is achieved.

5. Serve chilled.

Green Kiwi Juice

Ingredients: 2 kiwis, 1 cup fresh spinach leaves, 2 teaspoons honey, 1/2 cup water

Steps:

1. Peel and cut the kiwis into small pieces.

2. Add the kiwi cubes, fresh spinach leaves and honey to a blender.

3. Blend until smooth.

4. Add water and blend again until desired consistency is achieved.

5. Serve chilled.

CONCLUSION

In conclusion, Juicing for Beginners is an excellent resource for anyone interested in exploring the world of juicing. With its comprehensive coverage of ingredients, recipes, techniques, and nutrition, this book is sure to have something for everyone. Whether you are looking to make healthier food choices, lose weight, or just enjoy the benefits of juicing, you can be sure that this book will provide the information and inspiration you need to get started. With its easy-to-follow instructions and helpful advice, Juicing for Beginners is the perfect guide to jumpstart your journey into the world of juicing!